I0787524

HERBAL TREATMENT FOR THE MOST COMMON DISEASES

HERBAL TREATMENT

Medicinal plants, which have been a cure for many diseases for centuries, have become a cure for almost every disease, especially with the increase in science and technology, and research in the 21st century. There is no disease for which herbal treatments and methods to be applied after the required amount and dosage are determined by the experts. Considering that the essence of all medicinal drugs used today plants, the fact that herbal treatment methods are valid once again becomes clear. However, the lack of chemical side solutions in herbal treatment methods, as in most drugs, makes the treatment with herbs also important.

At this point, we can easily say this. By means of prescriptions prepared under the supervision of herbalists, provided that the priority is of course the specialist medical doctors; Many diseases such as heart, urinary tract, blood pressure, and diabetes can definitely be eliminated.

In this section of our book, you will find which herbal remedies can be applied and which diseases can cure.

HEALTH IN PLANTS

ABOUT HEALING PLANTS

The treatment of important diseases must be done by specialist doctors. However, in every minor ailment, the person may not need to be under medical supervision immediately. This book we have prepared will help you in this regard. It will introduce you to the plants, inform them about their activity forms and invite you to collect and dry the plants from nature with your own hands. In the meantime, it will often warn you about the details and limits of self-treatment with herbal teas. Herbal teas and tinctures are effective and harmless drugs. But in major diseases, they can only accompany or support the treatment of a specialist.

The person who wants to take care of herbs must have some basic knowledge about the plant's structure, organs, and functions. The various organs of a plant contain a variety of dissimilar active ingredients. In the field of treatment with herbs, these organs are defined as herbal drugs. Commonly used organs are leaves containing glycosides and alkaloids. Stems, which can be defined as a way of carrying between roots and leaves, are not generally used, but this rule may change in some plants. That is, the stems of some plants may also contain active ingredients. Likewise, the bark of some trees is rich inactive ingredients. The underground shoots, which act as a warehouse, according to their forms; Identified by the names rhizome, tuber, root, or onion. Roots send the water and mineral salts they absorb from the soil to the leaves. They usually store sugar, sometimes vitamins, and alkaloids. Flowers and fruits undertook the task of maintaining the lineage of the plant.

Generally, due to the active ingredients they contain, they have an important place in the field of treatment with herbs. The uncollected flower forms fruit. The plant seed is a storehouse containing the essence of the active ingredients necessary in the development stage of the plant. Stunted plants without flowers produce yellowish powders, similar to pollen.

In this book, generally recognized herbs and their therapeutic properties will be introduced that do not contain any side effects or toxic substances. With the information in this book, you can apply the prescriptions that you believe will be useful for you, with peace of mind. Sometimes it may be that you don't get positive results. However, you can absolutely believe that if you follow the recommended prescriptions properly and in the dosage, you will not get a bad result.

Dear readers, you may believe in the therapeutic power of medicinal herbs and even have achieved successful results with them. But if you value your health, do not neglect to see a doctor, especially for diseases that can have significant consequences! Symptoms that you consider to be simple ailments may be preliminary signs of a viral illness! Diagnosis and treatment of diseases can only be carried out by specialist medical doctors! Please do not ignore this issue and know that the priority regarding health is always with specialist medical doctors.

Take advantage of the therapeutic power of medicinal herbs to ward off your simple ailments. During the medical treatment of important diseases, you can support this treatment with herbs, with the approval of your doctor. But never attempt to treat yourself with herbs you don't know very well! Many medicinal plants in nature can cure all diseases, but scientific training is definitely needed to use these plants properly!

MENSTURAL PAIN

<u>Banana</u>: Thanks to the high amount of vitamin B6 it contains, it greatly reduces women's menstrual pain. It is like a natural pain reliever.

<u>Cinnamon</u>: It prevents the growth of Koli bacilli. When you drink lemon tea with honey, it is good for both sore throats caused by colds and menstrual pain.

LUNG DISEASES

Nettle seeds, black pepper, myrrh, honey, and mustard are mixed in equal amounts and eaten one tablespoon each morning and evening.

ALLERGY

<u>Apricot</u>: The substance called betacarotene prevents cancer by controlling molecules that attack cells. The brighter an apricot is, the higher the ratio of beta-carotene in it. Its calcium and magnesium content prevents larynx burns. Sulfur dioxide added to dried apricots is good for allergies such as asthma.

Treatments:

1- 100gr. nettle + 100gr. It is necessary to brew the horsetail mixture like tea, drink 3 tea glasses a day and continue this treatment for at least 20 days.

2- Falcon grass can be brewed like tea and drink 1 cup in the morning and evening.

3- A tablespoon of Bitter Chip and Ravend china is brewed and one glass is drunk in the morning and evening.

4- A pinch of chamomile is put in 1 tea glass of hot water and after a while, it is massaged into the eye by straining it. This treatment is repeated every 2 hours for 5-10 minutes.

APPENDICITIS

The most effective thing to prevent this disease is Blackberry tea.

VEHICLE HANDLING

<u>Ginger:</u> Helps digestion. It relieves nausea. It increases your energy. It reduces nausea and discomfort caused by traveling and driving for a long time.

ARPACIC MOUTH INJURIES

You can gargle with a mixture of vinegar and sesame oil. You can boil the mixture of one tablespoon of blackberry leaves, jujube, lentil, and edgy leaves and gargle while warm. You can mix raisins, anise and honey in the same amount and apply on the wounds. Chew a lot of thyme.

ARTIRITE

<u>Artichoke:</u> The biggest feature of artichokes is its ability to remove toxins. Therefore, it is especially recommended for patients with arthritis and rheumatism. A substance called Cynarine prevents the liver and gall bladder from becoming ill.

ASTHMA

<u>Onion:</u> Fights infections with garlic. Sulfur compounds prevent the arteries from being damaged. Onion; It is also good for bone resorption.

Treatments:

1- 1 lt. 1 pinch of myrtle leaf or nettle is put in water and boiled for 10 minutes and infused and filtered. 8-10 cups of tea a day are drunk without sugar.

2- 1 lt. 5 tablespoons of nettle are added to hot water, filtered after 5 minutes, and drink 8-10 glasses of sugar-free daily.

BOWEL

Apple: Helps digestion thanks to protein, vitamins, and natural chemicals. It facilitates digestion. They are characterized as a balancing and normalizing food for people with intestinal problems.

TONSIL

Thyme mouthwash is very effective. Fish oil should be drunk.

HEMORRHOIDS

Zulumba and Peganum seeds are mixed in equal proportions and eaten 1 teaspoon in the morning on an empty stomach.

HEADACHE

Mint: Peppermint tea is perfect for relieving headaches. Thanks to the menthol and menthol natural oils it contains, it also has the effect of relaxing the stomach.

Rosemary: It acts as a natural pain reliever thanks to its chemical ingredients.

Chocolate: It has natural antidepressant properties. Chocolate contains magnesium and iron. Thanks to its nervous relaxation feature, it relieves headaches.

Treatments:

There can be many causes of headaches. These reasons should be eliminated for effective treatment.

A pinch of lavender, chamomile, mint, rosemary, and thyme are added to 1 glass of hot water, filtered after 5 minutes, and drink 2-4 glasses a day.

KIDNEY AND BLADDER STONE

1 lt. A pinch of Horsetail, Corn Stigma, and Cherry stalk are put into the water, boiled for 5 minutes, and then filtered and drink 2-4 glasses a day.

To relieve pain; 1 lt. A pinch of flaxseed and licorice root are put in water, boiled for 15 minutes, and filtered and 3-4 glasses a day are drunk on an empty stomach.

SKIN PROBLEMS

Chamomile: Contains vegetable oil and chemicals. When drunk as a tea, it helps digestion and relieves abdominal pain. Chamomile tea bags to be prepared after a hot bath will relieve itching and burning caused by eczema.

Hot chili pepper: Contains 3 times more vitamin C than an orange. The chemical substance called Capsanthin is used in creams made to relieve pain caused by shingles.

Orange juice: A glass of orange juice provides your daily vitamin C needs.

meets all. The potassium in it maintains the body's water balance; It prevents skin drying and wrinkles.

Orange oil: When mixed with sesame oil, good skin oil is obtained. Also; It is recommended to massage the areas with cellulite with orange oil.

Treatment

80 gr. Rhubarb china is mixed with 1kg of honey and 1 dessert spoon is eaten on an empty stomach for 3 meals a day.

CELIAC DISEASE

Chestnut: It is an important source of energy. It can be easily digested. It can be a source of wheat-free flour for celiac patients. It contains vitamins E and B6 and is low in fat.

VESSEL OBSTACLE

250 gr. Chaste seed is boiled in 6 lt water for half an hour and 3 meals a day, one tea glass on an empty stomach (It has a blood pressure-lowering effect).

DEPRESSION

Avocado: This fruit is very easy to digest, especially for newborns.

We recommend it as the first food for babies. The vitamin E it contains is good for the heart, high potassium keeps it vigorous and beats the drowsiness and comfort that make people depressed. Adjusts the body's cholesterol ratio. It causes your skin to constantly renew cells. (Those who want to lose weight beware: We recommend that you do not eat avocados that are as high as chocolate fat).

Chocolate: Choose milk chocolate. Because the cocoa butter, magnesium, and vitamin E it contains help the brain to renew itself and provide psychological comfort. Those with migraines should stay away from chocolate.

Oyster: The iron in it increases the sperm count and the sex power of the human. Contains vitamins A, B12, and C. Clams, the most beneficial food for the brain, provide energy (Attention: Cholesterol ratio is twice that of many fish).

Potato: A medium potato contains the vitamin C a person should get in a day. It allows the chemical substance in the brain called serotonin to renew itself.

TOOTH

Bread: When sugary food is eaten, the acids in it attack the teeth every 20 minutes. Bread protects teeth. Eat 6 to 11 slices of bread throughout the day.

Fruit: (All kinds) Eat 2 to 4 meals a day.

Vegetables: (All kinds) Consume 3 to 5 meals a day.

Yogurt or feta cheese: If you think about your dental health while snacking between meals, choose these two foods that are rich in calcium.

Banana: Contains high amounts of carbohydrates. It is a rich source of potassium. This mineral ensures that the heart works regularly and blood pressure is regular.

DIABETES

Dry beans: It is a food rich in fiber. This greatly reduces the risk of diabetes. It takes a long time for the body to convert the carbohydrates it contains into sugar.

Lentil: Contains B vitamins, iron, calcium, potassium, phosphorus, and magnesium. Thanks to its soluble fiber, it reduces the cholesterol rate in the blood. For this reason, it is an indispensable food for diabetes and heart patients.

Cracked lips

Beeswax and rose oil are melted together and applied to the cracks. Sesame oil is also a good preservative.

Stomach Discomfort

Cinnamon: Relieves heartburn and vomiting.

Coconut: When added to milk drinks, it creates an effect of relaxing and gasifying the stomach. It prevents nausea.

<u>Cabbage:</u> Produces lactic acid during fermentation. This helps digestion by killing harmful bacteria in the digestive system.

ADOLESCENT CIVILS

It is useful to boil alum and narcissus in vinegared water and wipe the acne with this water.

PARALYSIS

<u>Citrus fruits:</u> Vitamin C rich citrus fruits prevent damage to the arteries and heart with the antioxidants called flavonoids they contain. The folic acid, heart-friendly potassium, and calcium contained in oranges cause healthy red blood cells to proliferate.

<u>Anchovy:</u> There is plenty of Omega-3s that reduce cholesterol and prevent blood clotting.

GASTRITIS

It is beneficial to drink a quarter of a teaspoon of mustard seeds with warm water every day before breakfast and to do this treatment as a 20-day cure.

EYE

<u>Corn:</u> Contains a herbal compound called Zeaxanthin. This substance reduces age-related visual impairment.

<u>Spinach:</u> Contains beta-carotene, which turns into vitamin A, which has antioxidant properties. It is necessary for healthy eyes. It also contains lutein substance against cataracts and deterioration of other eye layers. Consume immediately after cooking; In case of waiting, beneficial substances may turn into toxic substances.

FLU

<u>Satsuma (Small Orange):</u> Thanks to the folic acid and vitamin C it contains, it cuts cough and bloody saliva. In addition, since it is the

most effective natural food against blood clotting, it also reduces the risk of stroke or heart attack in advanced ages.

Cinnamon: It prevents the spread of E-coli bacteria that may have entered meals. It regulates the stomach. It prevents vomiting. It even cuts throat burning when taken with honey or lemon juice.

Mustard: The sinigrin substance in it helps the stomach to gas. It regulates the digestive system and relieves stomach pains. Maximum one teaspoon should be taken.

Mint: The menthol it contains causes normalization of the stomach. It fights against influenza germs that enter the body and also reduce the risk of getting ulcers in advanced ages. Peppermint tea is perfect for heartburn as well as diseases such as headache, flu, stress.

GOITER

It is mixed with butter seeds, seizure sugar, or honey in equal proportions and eaten. The sea sponge is cut into powder and mixed with honey and eaten.

GOUT (DROP DISEASE)

Anchovy: It is rich in omega-3 oil. It lowers the cholesterol level. By preventing blood clotting, it reduces the risk of vascular occlusion, heart attack, and therefore stroke. It is necessary to eat at least once a week. For heart patients, this amount should be 3-4 servings a week.

PREGNANCY

Artichoke: Contains plenty of folic acid and potassium. Low fat rate,

Thanks to its digestive effect and antioxidant properties, it has important benefits for the health of the mother and baby.

Blackberry: Contains vitamin E. It cleans harmful food waste in the body. Vitamin C is abundant. It protects the fetus.

HEMORRHOID

Coconut: The substance called myristin that it contains prevents vomiting, hemorrhoids.

(Caution! However, too much is dangerous for hemorrhoids).

URETHRA

Mint: It has diuretic properties. The menthol contains causes the normal function of the stomach. It fights against influenza germs that enter the body and also reduce the risk of getting ulcers in advanced ages. It stops nausea in the morning. Peppermint tea is perfect for heartburn as well as illnesses such as headaches and stress. However, drink mint tea on a full stomach, not on an empty stomach.

Apple: Vitamin C and pectin in it are very useful. It lowers cholesterol, regulates the digestive system, and eliminates problems in the urinary and urinary tract.

Whole wheat bread: Contains vitamin B3, iron, potassium, and folic acid. While too much of it damages the urinary tract, eating 2 slices a day is good.

HEART

Peas: A man who eats 10 servings of tomato peas a week has a 35 percent lower risk of developing prostate cancer than a person who does not. Peas, which are rich in B vitamins and protein, are also very important for the heart.

Whole Wheat Bread: It is beneficial for heart diseases and bowel cancer. More than 120 grams per day can be harmful to the individual.

Cherry: There are 40 calories in 100 grams. The ellagic acid it contains protects the body against cancer and ensures normal blood circulation in the cherry heart vessels. Eating too many cherries also reduces the risk of getting gout. Eating 20 cherries a day replaces 1 aspirin.

Chocolate: Vitamin E, magnesium, and iron; It reduces the risk of developing heart diseases. Eat a maximum of 1 chocolate per day.

Apple: Eat 5 a day.

Corn Flakes: 1 plate a day is enough.

Cucumber: Cucumber, which is the biggest help of dieters, lowers cholesterol. It strengthens the heart. Let's add without forgetting. Eat the salad without peeling it. Because the substance that strengthens the heart is between its shell and skin.

Egg: Contains the highest quality protein among all foods. Its most important feature is that it contains a lecithin substance that regulates cholesterol ratio. We recommend the egg cooked in a little oil in the pan.

Garlic: Don't miss out on your kitchen. Using at least 1000 natural remedies, garlic is beneficial for everything from the digestive system, cancer, blood circulation to heart diseases. But pregnant women should be careful. Excessive garlic also causes heartburn and palpitations. One tooth a day is enough.

Hummus: Rich in vitamin E, hummus also adjusts the blood cholesterol ratio.

Melon: Half of a melon meets all of the daily vitamin C needs of the human body and 15 percent of vitamin A. Melon is a frequently used fruit in the diets of heart and kidney patients.

Milk: A complete calcium, protein, folic acid, and phosphorus with vitamins A, E, and D store. It is recommended that children, young people, and pregnant women drink at least half a liter of milk a day.

Peach: One peach meets half your daily vitamin C needs. Choose the dark color of the fruit that is easy to digest. Because the betacarotene substance, which gives color to the shell, is beneficial against heart and cancer.

Rice: Contains all B vitamins except E and B12 and potassium. It is especially beneficial against colon and intestinal cancers. It is good for the heart as it lowers cholesterol.

Salt: It regulates the blood circulation and nervous system in the body. It is one-on-one for stomach cancer, osteoporosis, and heart problems. The British Ministry of Health announced to its people that 9 grams of salt per day is sufficient, and that excess will harm the body.

Tea: With 2 glasses of tea a day, you will get heart-friendly antioxidants such as 4 apples, 5 onions, 7 oranges. The British especially recommend that children drink at least 6 glasses of tea with milk per week.

Tuna Fish: Regulates cholesterol and blood pressure. Contains vitamin D and B12 against anemia. It protects the body against many cancers with the nicotinic acid it contains. A can of tuna meets the body's full vitamin D needs.

Turkey Meat: 125 grams of it meets the daily folic acid need of the body. Folic acid helps regenerate blood cells.

Watermelon: You meet 80% of your daily vitamin C needs with a slice. The potassium it contains provides blood circulation.

HEART ATTACK

Drinking Mistletoe tea, Melisa tea, and Sage has a preventive effect on the pot crisis. Also useful in Yarrow, Horsetail, and Thyme.

CANCER

Apricot: It is rich in beta-carotene which is an antioxidant. To cells and

It has a protective effect against cancer by removing the effect of molecules that damage tissues. Because it is fibrous, it protects the intestines.

Grains: Grains such as barley, corn, wheat, oats contain vitamins B and E, potassium, and calcium. It accelerates the process of removing carcinogenic substances from the body. A grain-based diet cuts the risk of bowel cancer in half.

Beans: Beans are rich in antioxidants such as vitamin C and beta-carotene that prevent heart disease and cancer. Vitamin B also strengthens sex hormones.

Beet: Being rich in iron and folic acid, beet has been used in the treatment of blood diseases since ancient times. American experts state that beet juice is also effective in the treatment of jaundice.

Cabbage: Contains carotene substance that prevents cancer cells from multiplying.

Carrots: 40 studies have revealed that the more carrot consumption increases, the lower the risk of cancer. The main reason for this is that it is rich in antioxidants such as beta-carotene, vitamins C and E.

Chickpea: Chickpea calcium with low-fat level and free of cholesterol,

It is rich in magnesium, phosphorus, potassium, copper, manganese, beta-carotene, and folic acid. It protects against breast cancer.

Fig: Contains potassium, iron, and calcium. It helps the digestive system. Used in the treatment of cancerous cells in ancient times, a fig is recommended by modern medicine as a protection against cancer.

Garlic: It strengthens the immune system and has a protective effect against cancer, high cholesterol, heart, and circulatory system diseases.

Hazelnuts: It is one of the foods richest in vitamin E, which is protective against heart attack. A handful of hazelnuts eaten every day are protective against cancer and wrinkles.

Lentil: Contains B vitamins, iron, calcium, magnesium, phosphorus, and potassium. Its fibrous feature lowers the cholesterol rate in the blood and is useful for diabetes and heart patients.

Olive Oil: Its omega fatty acids keep the cholesterol level in the blood in balance. It is also rich in vitamin E, which is an antioxidant. In this way, it has a protective effect on the brain against heart attack, stroke, cancer, and premature aging.

Onion: It strengthens the immune system. Contains allicin and sulfur; It has a protective effect against stomach and intestinal cancer. Recent studies have shown that it is more effective against osteoporosis than cheese and milk.

Peach: Even one can meet 50 percent of human vitamin C needs. It is easy to digest. It is also rich in beta-carotene, which is protective against cancer and heart attack. One has 33 calories.

Brass: Brass is an excellent source of energy. It is rich in vitamins E and B. Rice, which is protective against bowel cancer, reduces the risk of heart attack by lowering cholesterol.

Strawberry: It lowers the cholesterol level and regulates the digestive system. It also contains a carcinogenic substance called Ellagic acid.

Tomato: It is one of the rare plants rich in lycopene. Lycopene is vital in preventing various cancer diseases such as the pancreas. It is rich in vitamin C and strengthens the immune system. Being a fibrous food also reduces the risk of bowel cancer.

ANEMIA

Date: Although it varies according to the type, many dates contain high amounts of iron. They are an important source of energy with high nutritional value. It has a natural laxative effect. It contains a higher percentage of water and lower calories than dried ones.

Treatment

50 g. Henna, 1kg of black raisins and 1 / 2kg of plum, in 3lt of water

boiled for a while and drink 3 meals a day.

LIVER

Artichoke: Thanks to the substance called Cynarine, it helps the digestion of even the hardest foods. We strongly recommend those who suffer from rheumatism, arthritis, and gout, as well as pregnant women.

Licorice root: Many tribes around the world have used licorice root as a "natural remedy" for centuries against ulcers, arthritis, bronchitis, and liver ailments. It raises adrenaline, prevents people from being stressed, lowers blood pressure.

Turmeric: Aids digestion as well as liver ailments.

Abdominal pain

Chamomile tea: It removes the gas collected in the intestinal tract, regulates the digestive system, and cuts stomach pain.

MUSCULAR DYSTROPHY

3-4 glasses of Lion's Mane tea should be drunk in sips a day.

OSTEOCLASIS

<u>Apricot:</u> Contains high levels of calcium and magnesium.

<u>Milk:</u> It is a source of calcium, protein, vitamins B2-A-E-D, folic acid, phosphorus, and iron. It works together with calcium, vitamin D, and phosphorus to strengthen bones and teeth. Lack of these melts bones.

Treatment

3-4 glasses of Yarrow tea a day should be drunk in sips.

WEIGHT LOSS

<u>Chocolate pudding:</u> In this way, the blood in the body gets the protein and minerals it wants. The British Ministry of Health recommends that people who experience weight loss eat pudding 3 times a day for 1 week.

<u>Cheese:</u> There are 78 calories in 100 grams.

<u>Eggs:</u> 2 eggs a day meet 1 in 4 of the daily protein need of women and 1 in 5 of men. The selenium substance in the egg, which contains vitamins A, D, E, and B, solves digestive problems in babies and protects adults against cancer.

<u>Ice Cream:</u> Eating 2 balls of vanilla ice cream a day meets 20 percent of the daily protein requirement of the human body.

<u>Salami:</u> It is a source of B vitamins, iron, sodium, and potassium.

CALCIFICATION

400 g. Juniper seeds are mixed with 1kg of honey and 1 teaspoon of this mixture is eaten 3 times a day on an empty stomach.

LACTOSE RESISTANCE

<u>Almond:</u> Contains high levels of calcium, magnesium, potassium, phosphorus, vitamin E, vitamin B2, antioxidants. For this reason,

almonds are an ideal food source for those who have lactose (milk sugar) weakness and cannot eat daily foods.

MENOPAUSE

Chickpea: Contains vegetable hormone "phytoestrogen". These are the effects of estrogen in the body

balance its effects and protects against the effects of menopause. It is one of the richest sources of vegetable protein.

Cola: Caffeine relieves body fatigue and provides concentration.

Grape: Thanks to the "pelagic" acid it contains, the bone caused by menopause

protects against melting. It also minimizes menopausal symptoms by increasing the level of estrogen in the blood.

Prunes: Even just two or three meals meet the antioxidants the body needs. It relaxes the urinary tract muscles. This protects against colon cancer. It contains iron, vitamin A, vitamin B6, and potassium. Thanks to the high rate of boron mineral it contains, it keeps the estrogen level in balance in women during menopause.

Sweet potato: It provides energy to the body by strengthening the adrenal glands. It contains phosphorus, magnesium, calcium, vitamin C, potassium, and folic acid.

SHORTNESS OF BREATH

Some Sea kadayıf is pulverized. 1 teaspoon in linden

It is boiled and drunk by adding it in proportion.

COUGH

Laurel seed is mixed with honey and eaten, provided that it is not more than 20 grams per day. 100 gr. powdered ginger and 100 gr.

Powdered turmeric is mixed with 1kg of honey and eaten 3 times a day on an empty stomach and 1 dessert spoon.

PROSTATE

100 g. Boil the root in 5 liters of water until 2.5 liters remain. 3 meals a day, half an hour before meals, 1 tea glass is drunk. The same amount of celery seeds is prepared in the same way and 1 tea glass is drunk 3 times a day, 15 minutes before meals.

RHEUMATISM

Artichoke: Thanks to its effect of removing the poison in the body, it is perfect against rheumatism, gout disease, and joint burning. Folic acid and potassium strengthen bones.

Tomato: Vitamin C is abundant.

Cereal: The natural chemicals it contains relieve joint burns and rheumatic pain caused by rheumatism.

Thyme: A type of natural oil called thymol allows other fats in the body to break down. When thyme oil is applied in the bath, it greatly reduces rheumatism pain.

Ginger: Its stimulant effects dilate blood vessels and increase blood circulation, eliminating rheumatism pain and burning.

Treatments:

1- Mustard seeds are beaten and mixed with honey and eaten. Also, it is applied to the painful area.

2- The following oils are mixed in certain proportions and applied to the painful area.

Balsam oil: 100 gr.

Oregano oil: 70 gr.

Trout oil: 50 gr.

Clove oil: 25 gr.

PSORIASIS

50 gr. Nettle, 50 gr. Basil and 50 gr. Yarrow 1 lt. Keep it in hot water for 15 minutes, strain it and drink 3-4 glasses a day.

DIGESTIVE PROBLEMS

Barley: Minerals such as calcium and potassium, and vitamin B, give the body resistance. In addition, a study in the USA has proven that eating barley products every day for 6 months reduces cholesterol by 15 percent.

Yogurt: 150 grams of yogurt a day increases the daily calcium requirement of the body.

meets. Since 3 teaspoons of sugar are added to fruit yogurts, their sugar ratio is higher. The potassium in yogurt regulates blood pressure and heart rate. It allows the stomach to grind food regularly.

CYSTITIS

Asparagus: Contains folic acid, vitamins C and E. It helps to remove the toxic residues of the food in the body. It facilitates and supports the work of the liver and kidneys. That's why doctors say cystitis patients should definitely eat asparagus.

STRESS

Mayan root: Has an antivirus effect. It protects the liver. It balances the secretion of adrenaline. It releases cortisol hormone, which is necessary to cope with stress.

DIABETES

1 lt. 20 g in hot water. Put the myrtle leaf and infuse for 5-10 minutes and drink it throughout the day. 250 gr. cypress cones, 250 gr. wormwood and 100 gr. lemon balm 2.5 lt. put into alcohol. It is

kept in an airtight container for 45 days and drunk 3 times a day, on an empty stomach, by adding 8-10 drops to 1 coffee cup in water.

BLOOD PRESSURE

Fennel: Thanks to the potassium it contains, it regulates blood pressure. It also contains plenty of folic acids, which is essential for healthy blood cells. Fennel tea is good for digestion.

Grain: It contains a kind of photosynthetic chemical that relaxes and relaxes blood vessels. In this way, it enables the blood to pass through the veins more easily. Eating grains allows more calories to be burned in the body than vegetables. The reduction in calories regulates blood pressure.

Flour: It contains the nutritional values of the grain from which it is made. It is rich in B vitamins, vitamin E, iron, and magnesium.

Liver: It is rich in vitamin A, which is essential for a healthy immune system, skin, and sharp eyes. A small portion provides daily vitamin A and iron and monthly vitamin B12 needs.

THYROID

Mussels: It is a rich food source in terms of Omega-3 oil. The selenium mineral it contains is necessary for the normal functioning of the thyroid glands.

ULCER

Cabbage: For people with ulcers, it creates a tonic, that is, stomach cleansing effect. It contains high levels of vitamin C. Red cabbage contains vitamin A, which has antioxidant properties in the body. It has an anti-cancer effect. It is recommended to be added to salads raw.

IF THE BODY HAS to HOLD WATER

Currant: 100 grams of it meets exactly 3 times the daily vitamin C requirement. It has antibacterial and anti-burning effects. Its rich potassium and low salt content is an important natural remedy for those with dehydration.

Zucchini: 100 grams of pumpkin meets one-fourth of the daily folic acid need. The high percentage of potassium provides the liquid-salt balance.

Grain: People with dehydration disorders should definitely eat thanks to its opening, activating, and relaxing effects on the urinary tract. It has a relaxing feature on the stomach.

SIMPLE TREATMENT METHODS WITH VEGETABLES AND FRUITS

HEALING IN VEGETABLES AND FRUITS

Sage: It removes stomach and intestinal gas. It stops nausea. It provides a regular digestive system. It softens the breast. It is useful for asthma patients.

Raspberry: Cleans the blood, removing toxic substances accumulated in the body

provides. It makes you sweat and diuretic. It relieves constipation. It gives vigor to the body.

Anise: It facilitates digestion. Lack of appetite and food

removes disgust. Stomach and intestinal gas are removed. Increases urine. On the other hand, prevent vomit and diarrhea.

Vine: Medicines made with leaves stop bleeding. It gives strength to the body. Cuts yellowness. It stops diarrhea.

Avocado: Although it is very calorie, the Glutathione it contains is a supercell protector because it is the best antioxidant. Antioxidants slow down the aging of cells and prevent cancer. It is the richest in protein among all fruits. It also contains plenty of vitamin E. This vitamin protects the heart and the skin and improves circulation. It also contains potassium and vitamin B6. It is very necessary for women.

Split grass: It is a diuretic. Kidney and helps reduce bladder stones. It also removes inflammations in these areas.

Quince: It cuts diarrhea and dysentery. It strengthens the stomach and intestines. It relieves small intestine inflammation. It cleans the blood. It relieves palpitations.

Walnut: Medicines prepared with leaves and shells clean the blood and removes anemia. It cuts diarrhea and dysentery. It is both nutritious and therapeutic in tuberculosis and diabetes. Also used to dye hair and hands. According to herbalists, walnuts, which contain plenty of vitamins A, B1, B2, C, E, and K and an active ingredient called Chinon Juglone, are good for many health problems. Eating some walnuts at breakfast every morning improves intelligence, and when boiled and drunk green walnut shells, it increases sexual power in men. Some of the benefits of walnuts, which nourish and strengthen the body, are listed as follows:

• Walnut oil put on the calluses will make them disappear over time.

• The liquid obtained by mixing and boiling with the shells of fresh branches and fruit shells strengthens the stomach.

• Tea made from walnut leaves increases appetite, strengthens the stomach, and is good for throat diseases.

• If some walnut leaves are mixed into the bathwater, it is good for skin diseases.

• If walnut leaves are wrapped on boils by cooking, they will heal them.

• If walnut oil is rubbed on the face stains and massaged, the stains will disappear.

Pistachio: Bronchitis, tuberculosis, rapid recovery of lung diseases

It helps. It removes the spiritual depression. It is also useful in heart diseases.

Fenugreek : It removes sputum. It gives comfort to the body.

Strawberry: Fresh and juicy strawberries clean the system. it is a good fruit for people who have skin condition too. It is also good for kidney, urinary tract, and intestinal problems. It also strengthens the gums, prevents tartar in the teeth, and eliminates mouth odor and sore throats. Strawberries contain high levels of vitamin C, as well as substances that reduce high blood pressure and cholesterol. Strawberry meets the vitamin C need. It also contains plenty of potassium and takes an important place among fiber foods. Diabetic patients can eat this fruit a lot, provided that they do not add sugar to the strawberry.

Black seed: It increases appetite. It gives strength and vigor to the body. It facilitates digestion. It removes stomach and intestinal gases. Cuts headaches if you smelled.

Laurel: Makes sweat, reduces fever. It gives comfort to the body. It removes urine and menstruation. It increases appetite. It relieves nerve pain.

Sea Kadayıf: It removes respiratory and digestive system colds. Used as a feeder body.

Seaweed: It speeds up the functioning of metabolism. Seaweed containing substances that prevent imbalances in thyroid hormone speeds up the metabolism. Also, algae containing B vitamins, calcium, and zinc; Effective against skin, nails, and hair.

Thistle: Reduces fever. It makes you sweat and gives comfort to the body.

Tomato: A vegetable that prevents cancer and slows down aging mentally and physically. Contains vitamins C and E. Tomatoes are a rich source of potassium and a very little salt. It helps to reduce high blood pressure and prevents the body from water retention. effective against prostate cancer and heart disease. 'It contains lycopene which is close to beta carotene. Lycopene is among the substances that protect the body against heart diseases. Searches indicate that tomato reduces the risk of cancer. Men who eat tomatoes at least twice a week have less risk of developing prostate cancer than others.

Mulberry: White mulberry leaves are diuretic. It drains the water accumulated in the body. White mulberry eaten on an empty stomach intestinal worms are removed.

Mallow: Softens the breast. Cough stops. Prevents nausea and vomiting. It reduces fever and gives comfort to the body. It removes throat and tonsillitis. It treats gum disease.

Apple: Eating an apple a day keeps the doctor away from your home. If you eat two apples, you will be protected against heart and circulation problems. It removes cholesterol and prevents constipation. It facilitates digestion. It relieves odor and lowers blood pressure. It is also useful against arthritis, rheumatism, and gout.

Artichoke: It lowers urea and cholesterol in the blood. It is a diuretic. Adjusts the amount of sugar in the blood. It prevents arteriosclerosis and heart diseases. It helps to pour the sand into the kidney.

Important: It is good against prostate, breast, and cervical cancer.

Pointing out that the Silymarin substance in the artichoke prevents the cells from being damaged, the researchers also stated that the Silymarin substance is also effective in preventing prostate, breast, and cervical cancer. It has been found that artichokes contain fiber, magnesium, folate, and vitamin C, and those who consume this vegetable in large quantities show less than their age.

Basil: It stops coughing. It stops dizziness. In bee sting is useful. It treats mouth sores. Basil scent, mosquito and repels insects such as bedbugs.

Hazelnut: It removes body and mind fatigue. It gives strength to the body. The recovery circuit enables you to move quickly.

Poppy: Provides relief in shortness of breath, asthma, and bronchitis. Prevents coughing and vomiting blood. It heals burns.

Grapefruit: It is very rich in vitamin C. Half a grapefruit provides 60 percent of the daily vitamin C requirement. It contains a pectin substance that lowers the cholesterol ratio. It has a protective feature against cancer. It increases appetite.

Alcea: It heals mouth, throat, and gingivitis. Intestinal inflammations fixes.

Carrots: If eaten five times a week, it reduces the risk of heart infarction and stroke by 68 percent in women, according to Harvard's research. Two carrots a day have been shown to reduce blood cholesterol by 10 percent in men. A carrot is eaten every day also cuts the risk of lung cancer in half. Beta-Carotene in carrots also protects the eyes from vision weakness caused by old age and strengthens the immune system. It prevents stomach and intestinal bleeding, removes anemia, increases breast milk, removes face and neck wrinkles, removes urine and intestinal gas, eliminates ulcer complaints. As it is effective against cancer, it also prevents drying of the skin and strengthens the immune system. One of the greatest properties of carrot, which contains beta carotin (stops cancer-causing free radicals and strengthens the immune system), is that this substance can turn into vitamin A, which prevents skin from drying.

Date: The magic power of the apple in protection from cardiovascular diseases was known until today. Israeli scientists proved to be a true friend of palm heart. Israeli scientists explained that dates are more effective than apples recommended for preventing cardiovascular diseases. In a study conducted in Israel, the benefits of apples and dates were compared. Date; Scientists, who say that it is rich in fiber, minerals, and phenols, stated that there is more copper and zinc in apples, whereas the amounts of sodium, potassium, magnesium, calcium, and iron in dates are twice as high. Scientists have noted that the beneficial substances in these fruits, which reduce the risk of cardiovascular diseases if eaten regularly, are mostly found in their peels.

Nettle: When applied externally, it draws blood accumulated in internal organs. It stops nosebleeds. It removes phlegm.

Spinach: It is an effective vegetable against heart diseases, stroke, high blood pressure, eye diseases caused by old age, cancer, and even psychic disorders. Eye diseases and effective against staining of the skin. Spinach is effective against vision disorders thanks to the two chemicals it contains. It shows that 86 percent of those who eat spinach 6 times a week will not have a problem such as staining on the skin that occurs with age. It is also effective against eye diseases that occur with age. One serving of spinach, covering one-tenth of our daily needs for iron.

Fig: Softens the intestines. It relieves constipation. It is good for bronchitis, coughs, and sore throats. It gives energy.

Clove: It kills germs. It relieves pain. It stimulates the nerves. It facilitates digestion. It removes the odor. It increases appetite.

Thyme: It strengthens the body. It facilitates digestion. It cuts heart palpitations. It heals intestinal inflammations. It helps to reduce intestinal worms. It reduces the amount of sugar in the blood.

Red Pepper: Effective against infectious diseases. It increases the body's resistance to infectious diseases. This vegetable, which contains more vitamin C than an orange, also strengthens our immune system with the beta carotin it contains. 100 grams of dried red peppers provide 318 calories of energy, 148 milligrams of calcium, 76 milligrams of vitamin C (340 milligrams in fresh peppers), 8.1 grams of water, 2 thousand 14 milligrams of potassium, 41 thousand 610 IU of vitamin A, 12 grams of protein, 293 milligrams of phosphorus, It contains 15 milligrams of vitamin B3, 17.3 grams of fat, 152 milligrams of magnesium, 2 milligrams of vitamin B2, 56.6 grams of carbohydrates, 30 milligrams of sodium, 1 milligram of vitamin B1, 24.9 grams of fiber, 8 milligrams of iron, as well as organic compounds such as bitterness and coloring matter. It is a known fact that red pepper, which is of great importance in nutrition, is also a sought-after material in human health. Red pepper increases gastric juice and saliva formation, digestion It removes rheumatism, joint, and toothaches, removes cramps, is good for many diseases, especially cholera and gout. It reduces cancer risk and is used in cancer treatment. It increases sweating, gives coolness (this is one of the reasons why it is used in hot climates), is used to relieve cough and sore throat (as a mouthwash), it is a natural soothing for nervous diseases, it prevents the accumulation of excess fat and cholesterol in the body. Red pepper, which is also effective in preventing diseases with its antibacterial effect, is widely consumed in South and Southeastern provinces, mainly Kahramanmaraş, Gaziantep, and Şanlıurfa. The red peppers of this area are hot types. Red pepper is mostly produced in Bursa and Bilecik in the north. These peppers are usually sweet. Henna: Reduces fever. It treats malaria. Useful in typhoid. It increases appetite. It is useful in skin itching.

Cherry: Eating cherries are much more effective than aspirin in relieving pain. People living in the state of Michigan in the USA eat a lot of cherries as they grow a lot in this region. Some argue that this fruit is perfect for pain caused by gout and joint inflammation. Muraleedharan Nair from Michigan State University has been shown to have this effect of red chemicals known as "anthocyanin" in cherry. Points out that he can create. Using common experiments, Nair and his team investigated whether the compounds contained enzymes found in pain relievers such as aspirin and ibuprofen. He then examined the detrimental properties of chemicals from free radicals and compared them with vitamins. As a result, it was seen that there were 12-25 milligrams of anthocyanin in 20 cherries and the pain relief effect of this substance was 10 times more than aspirin. It was also witnessed that the anthocyanin substance contained in cherries had antioxidant effects similar to vitamins E and Ca. According to Nair, eating 20 cherries a day has the same effect as taking an aspirin. Nair is working on converting the anthocyanin in cherries to tablets.

Kiwi: A kiwi has twice the amount of vitamin C in an orange. They are also rich in potassium. Facilitate digestion and preventing constipation.

Rosehip: It is friendly to the eyes due to its very intense vitamin richness. Provides vitality to the body. 100 grams of rosehip contains vitamin C equivalent to a crate of orange. A good rickets remedy is an effective blood cleanser. It is a powerful worm reducer and intestinal softener. It is beneficial against stomach cramps and digestive system difficulties. It relieves rheumatism pain. It gives good results in the treatment of hemorrhoids. Asparagus: Effective against indigestion. Containing anti-toxic substances, this vegetable kidney purifies from toxins and facilitates the digestion of nutrients.

Cabbage : It is one of the vegetables known to be effective against cancer. It contains plenty of B, C, and E vitamins, potassium. It is especially effective against breast and uterine cancer. It provides the removal of toxic substances accumulated in the body. It lowers the amount of sugar in the blood. It is good for jaundice and gall bladder diseases. It is beneficial for asthma. It is effective against bowel cancer. Cabbage contains a chemical substance (isothiocyanates) that inhibits the growth of cancer cells. According to a study conducted in the USA, the risk of bowel cancer is reduced by two-thirds for those who eat cabbage once a week.

Parsley: There is no problem that parsley, the ornament of salads and meals, is almost not a cure. A storehouse of vitamins A and C and iron, sulfur, phosphorus, and manganese elements, parsley facilitates digestion, reduces kidney stones, increases vision and breast milk. It is an iron warehouse. Usually, fresh parsley contains calcium, potassium, and vitamin A. A pinch of parsley meets most of the daily vitamin C requirement. It brings urine by activating the kidneys and lowers stones, keeps blood sugar at a normal level, and is also protective against cancer. When eaten before bedtime allows us to wake up in the morning with a sweet breath. Increases breast milk. It throws out toxic substances from the body. Its eyesight increases, it is good for acne when it is boiled and smoked and the skin is dressed with this water. Boiled parsley juice prevents inflammation in the eyes when the eyes are dressed and pass burning. When the hair is boiled and washed with vinegar, it helps the hair grow and strengthen.

Mushroom: It strengthens the immune system. This vegetable, which the Chinese eat as medicine, protects the body against diseases and strengthens the immune system.

Lettuce: Effective against osteoporosis. This vegetable, which contains even more calcium than milk, is number one in terms of strengthening bones. At 100 grams, it has more calcium than a small glass of milk. This amount is equivalent to one-quarter of the daily calcium needs.

Angelica: It regulates blood circulation. It makes you sweat. If it is driven to kill head lice dried angelica beaten. It is beneficial for asthma attacks.

Licorice: It is beneficial for flu, cold, angina, and shortness of breath. It removes cough and phlegm. It lowers high blood pressure.

Corn: It contains high fiber, at 18.3 percent. High carbohydrate into the corn increases your energy level. It contains protein, calcium, iron, phosphorus, vitamins A and B2.

Banana: It is an extremely rich fruit in terms of folic acid, potassium, and vitamin B6. Potassium prevents cramps.

Pomegranate: It strengthens the body. Cuts diarrhea. It is beneficial for nasal polyps. It lowers sugar. It strengthens the heart. Those with stomach and intestinal diseases, young children, and pregnant women should not overuse.

Chickpea: It strengthens the body. Increases breast milk.

Mistletoe: Increases the heartbeat. It is useful in vascular calcification. It is used in epilepsy and lung bleeding.

Potato: If you don't eat fried, it won't gain weight. It facilitates digestion, prevents constipation. It is perfect against fatigue. It contains plenty of vitamin C and protein. The potato, which contains carbohydrates, which is the energizing substance for the body, is richest in vitamins C and E and beta carotene. 100 grams of potatoes have 80 calories, 2 grams of protein, 17 mg of carbohydrates, 7 mg of calcium, 53 mg of phosphorus, 20 mg of vitamin C. It's always said, it's okay if it's said one more time; Since most of the potato's nutritional value is in the skin, it is better to scrape it with a special knife rather than peel it. Potatoes cooked with the peel loses 25 percent of vitamin C. For this reason, it is necessary to cook the potato in the oven with its skin, or in steam or little water.

Leek: It is a diuretic. It is good for stomach discomfort. It relieves constipation. It is useful for hemorrhoids. It helps reduce the sand and stones in the kidney.

Orange: A fruit full of antioxidants. It includes all things which are known as an inhibitor for cancer. It also contains plenty of vitamin C. It prevents weight gain. It lowers cholesterol in the blood. The body reduces the risk of cancer with vitamin C, potassium, protein, B and E vitamins, heart diseases, and anticarcinogenic substances.

Cucumber: The cucumber itself or its water cleanses our skin as much as a tonic. Cucumber prevents constipation and helps to remove the water accumulated in the body in kidney and heart diseases. It is effective against heart diseases and infections. It contains sulfur and this substance increases the body's resistance to infections as well as lowers cholesterol.

Sahlep: It is beneficial for cough and bronchitis. It ensures regular menstrual bleeding. It increases the power to run the mind.

Onion and Garlic: They reduce the risk of high blood pressure and heart disease. Onion, the risk of stomach cancer; garlic also reduces the risk of developing bowel cancer. The substances in the yeast of garlic protect the body against premature aging by preventing damage to the cells. Garlic, which contains antibiotics and compounds that relieve shortness of breath, also strengthens the immune system. effective against heart and allergic diseases. Onion strengthens our hearts and prevents allergic reactions to the chemical substances it contains. Studies conducted in Newcastle show that those who regularly eat onions have a reduced risk of clogging their arteries.

Soy: Anyone who wants to live long should definitely consume soy. Soy contains a substance that functions similar to the estrogen hormone and dilutes the effects of this hormone, which is extremely beneficial for the female body. Because excessive production of estrogen hormone, which accelerates cell renewal, increases the risk of breast, uterine, and neck cancer.

Cinnamon: It relieves spiritual troubles. Useful in surveillance. It strengthens the heart. It increases appetite and facilitates digestion.

Cress: Appetite. It facilitates digestion. It cleans the bronchi and coughs. Diuretic cleanses the kidneys and urinary tract. It is effective against cancer, anemia, and fiber diseases. As it is among the vegetables that fight cancer, it is also one of the ones containing the most calcium, iron, and folic acid. Women who eat green vegetables such as cress have less risk of getting life-related diseases.

Tuna: Although it is very fatty, it contains an important fatty acid called Omega-3. This substance is good for high blood pressure, heart palpitations, and severe migraine pain. It also treats skin dryness and eczema. However, it should be eaten fresh. Canned tuna contains high vitamin D but lacks Omega-3 fatty acids.

Radish: Kills germs in the kidneys. It helps to pour sand and stones. It reduces liver swelling. It is useful for jaundice. It helps to reduce gallstones. it is good for rheumatism, asthma, and bronchitis.

Cherry: Cuts diarrhea. It reduces fever. It is diuretic. It gives comfort to the body.

Allspice: Prevents vascular stiffness. It facilitates digestion. It clears stomach and bowel gases.

Yogurt: Among the bacteria found in various organs of the body, the ones that live in the intestine are important for the regular functioning of the digestive system. These bacteria can be attacked by infections and the antibiotics we have to take when we have an infectious disease. This destroys the digestive system. Yogurt solves this problem, restores the reduced amount of bacteria to its normal level and both prevents and combats infections. It also stimulates the immune system. Yogurt, which has more calcium than milk, is equal to the protein ratio to milk.

Oats: It relieves the digestive difficulties of children. It removes physical and mental fatigue. It reduces the amount of sugar in the blood.

Jerusalem artichoke: It is useful for diabetics. It is nutritious. It increases the body's resistance. It relieves constipation.

Ginger: It increases appetite. It prevents vomiting. It removes intestinal disorders.

Olive: Olive oil increases bile. It works the liver. It cuts liver pain. It is useful for jaundice. Leaves and shells reduce high blood pressure. It lowers the amount of sugar in the blood. It helps to reduce intestinal worms.